MEDICATION CLASSES FOR NCLEX

A QUICK REFERENCE GUIDE FOR RN/PN

AMY PAINTER MSN, FNP

CONTENTS

INTRODUCTION

This guide has three sections to help you be successful on NCLEX pharmacology. Each section can assist you by itself, but together they can be an even more powerful tool to improve your grasp of common pharmacological concepts and drugs. With them, you can synthesize knowledge in a way that can increase recognition and knowledge about families or classes of drugs instead of trying to learn every commonly prescribed drug.

This guide is applicable to both RN and PN students. PN students may find that they may not give a certain route of a drug family, but still may care for a patient receiving a drug in that class by a different route.

The guide is split into three sections:

- Section 1 includes tables listing common prefixes and suffixes found in the names of generic medications.

- Section 2 lists an outline of the major drug classes and families. The outline includes a common or "gold standard" medication that can be easily referenced for more in depth study of that class. The way the outline is displayed helps one understand the hierarchy and associations of various classes.

- Section 3 includes NCLEX style questions and rationales on the drugs found in Section 1. This provides good practice for many of the families to be found on the NCLEX.

Section I

Pharmacological Prefix and Suffix Tables

The following tables include common prefixes and suffixes found in generic medications. When applicable, both the generic and trade name of a drug is referenced as such *generic name* (Trade name). Please be aware that a generic medicine can have multiple trade names. This is not meant to be an all-inclusive list. It is also not intended to market for any particular pharmaceutical.

Please do not infer that all drugs in that drug class have that prefix. There are many drug classes that have varied generic names. For example in the class of opioids, one does use the prefix "oxy" in oxycodone, and oxymorphone, however other drug names in that class include "mor" with hydromorphone and morphine sulfate.

Prefix	Drug Class/ Category	Examples: *generic name* (Trade name)
Cefa-, cepha-	Cephalosporin, Anti-infective	*cefazolin* (Ancef), *cefoxitin* (Mefoxin), *ceftriaxone* (Rocephin), *cephalexin* (Keflex)
Pre-, Pred-	Steroids	*prednisone* (Sterapred), *prednisolone* (Oraped)
Sulfa-	Anti-infective, Sulfonamides	*sulfadiazine, trimethoprim/ sulfamethoxazole* (Bactrim)
Mor-, -mor-	Opioids	*hydromorphone* (Dilaudid), *morphine sulfate* (MS Contin)
Oxy-	Opioids	*oxycodone* (OxyContin), *oxymorphone* (Opana)
Chole-, cole-	Bile Acid Sequestrants, Cardiovascular	*cholestyramine* (Questran), *colesevelam* (Welchol)
Est-	Estrogens, Endocrine	*estradiol vaginal* (Premarin), *estrogens esterified* (Estratest)
Progest-	Progestins, Endocrine	*progesterone* (Crinone), *medoxyprogesterone* (Provera)
Cort-	Endocrine, Corticosteroids	*cortisone, hydrocortisone* (Cortef)
Tretin-	Dermatology, Anti-cancerous	*tretinoin topical* (Retin-A), *isotretinoin* (Accutane), *Tretinoin ingested* (Vesanoid)

Section 1: Pharmacological Prefix and Suffix Tables

Suffix	Drug Class/ Category	Examples: *generic name* (Trade name)
-sone	Steroids Hormones, Endocrine	*prednisone, dexamethasone* (Decadron), *hydrocortisone* (Cortef), *fluticasone* (Flovent)
-lone	Steroid Hormones, Endocrine	*prednisolone* (Flo-Pred), *methylprednisolone acetate* (Depo-Medrol), *triamcinolone acetonide* (Trivaris)
-profen	NSAIDS, Anti-inflammatory	*ibuprofen* (Advil), *flurbiprofen* (Ansaid)
-cillin	Penicillin, Anti-infectives	*amoxicillin* (Amoxil), *penicillin, ampicillin/sulbactam* (Unasyn), *piperacillin/tazobactam* (Zosyn)
-cycline	Tetracyclines, Anti-infectives	*minocycline* (Minocin), *tetracycline* (Sumycin), *doxycyclin* (Vibramycin)
-caine	Anesthetic	*prilocaine, marcaine, lidocaine*
-nafil	Erectile Dysfunction, Genitourinary, Pulmonary arterial hypertension	*tadalafil* (Cialis), *vardenafil* (Levitra), *sildenafil* (Viagra)
-prazole	Proton pump inhibitors, Gastrointestional	*omeprazole* (Prilosec), *lansoprazole* (Prevacid), *esomeprazole* (Nexium)
-dipine	Calcium Channel Blockers, Cardiovascular	*amlodipine* (Norvasc), *nifedipine* (Adalat), *nicardipine* (Cardene),
-floxacin	Quinolone, Anti-infectives	*moxifloxacin* (Avelox), *ciprofloxacin* (Cipro), *levofloxacin* (Levaquin)

Medication Classes For NCLEX

-mycin	Macrolides, Anti-infectives	*clarithromycin* (Biaxin), *erthromycin* (EryPed), *azithromycin* (Zithromax, Zpack)
-azole	Anti-fungal, Anti-infective Antiparasitic, Anti-infective	*fluconazole* (Diflucan), *itracanazole* (Sporanox), *ketocanazole* *metronidazole* (Flagyl)
-lol	Beta Blockers, Cardiovascular	*atenolol* (Tenormin), *propranolol* (Inderal), *carvedilol* (Coreg)
-pril	ACE inhibitor, Antihypertensive	*captopril* (Capoten), *lisinopril* (Zestril), *enalapril* (Vasotec)
-sartan	ARB, Antihypertensive	*valsartan* (Diovan), *irbesartan* (Avapro), *losartan* (Cozaar)
-mide, -nide	Loop Diuretics, Cardiovascular	*bumeanide* (Bumex), *furosemide* (Lasix), *torsemide* (Demadex)
-setron	Anti-emetic, Gastrointestional	*ondansetron* (Zofran), *dolasetron* (Anzemet)
-statin	Anticholesterol Statins, Cardiovascular	*lovastatin* (Altoprev), *rosuvastatin* (Crestor), *fluvastatin* (Lescol)
-terol	Bronchodilator/Beta 2 Agonists	*albuterol sulfate* (Albuterol HFA), *formoterol* (Foradil), *salmeterol* (Serevent)
-thiazide	Thiazide Diuretics, Cardiovascular	chlorothiazide (Diuril), methylclothiazide, hydrochlorothiazide (Microzide)
-triptan	Anti-migraine, Neurological	*sumatriptan* (Alsuma), *naratriptan* (Amerge), *almotriptan* (Axert)
-vir	Antiviral	*ganciclovir* (Cytovene), *valacyclovir* (Valtrex), *acyclovir* (Zovirax), *oseltamivir* (Tamiflu)

-zepam, zolam	Benzodiazepines	*alprazolam* (Xanax), *midazolam* (Versed), *lorazepam* (Ativan), *temazepam* (Restoril), *clonazepam* (Klonopin)
-zosin	Alpha blocker, Cardiovascular	*doxazosin* (Cardura), *terazosin* (Hytrin), *prazosin* (Minipress)
-cin	Anti-infective, aminoglycosides	*amikacin* (Amikin), *neomycin sulfate, tobramycin* (Tobi)
-zolamide	Anti-infective, carbonic anhydrase inhibitors	*brinzolamide* (Azopt), *acetazolamide* (Diamox)
-ine	Antihistamines Also seen in Antiarrhythmics, Cardiovascular Also seen in immunosuppressants Also seen in Antidepressants/ SNRIs	*diphenhydramine* (Benadryl), *meclizine* (Antivert), *hydroxyzine* (Atarax), *loratadine* (Claritin), *fexofenadine* (Allegra), *adenosine* (Adenocard), *epinephrine* (Adrenalin), *atropine, dobutamine* *azathiprine* (Azasan), *cyclosporine* (Gengraf), *azathioprine* (Imuran) *duloxetine* (Cymbalta), *venlafaxine* (Effexor)
-ol	Opioids	*tramadol* (Ultram), *levorphanol* (Levo-Dromoran), *tapentadol* (Nucynta)
-ium	Neuromuscular Blockers	*vecuronium* (Norcuron), *pancuronium* (Pavulon), *cisatracurium* (Nimbex)
-penem	Carbapenems, anti-infectives	*ertapenem* (Invanz), *meropenem* (Merem), *doripenem* (Doribax)
-tropium	Anticholinergics, inhaled	*ipratropium bromide* (Atrovent), *tiotropium* (Spiriva)

-one	Antiarrhthmics, Cardiovascular	*amiodarone* (Pacerone), *dronedarone* (Multaq)
	Also seen in Steroid Hormones	*testosterone* (Androderm), *oxandrolone* (Oxandrin), *prednisone, methylprednisolone acetate* (Depo-Medrol)
-arin	Anticoagulants, Cardiovascular	*warfarin* (Coumadin), *fondaparinux* (Arixtra), *enoxaparin* (Lovenox)
-pi-	Antiplatelets, Cardiovascular	*aspirin, clopidogrel* (Plavix), *ticlopidine* (Ticlid)
-plase	Thrombolytics, Cardiovascular	*alteplase* (Activase), *reteplase* (Retavase), *tenecteplase* (TNKase)
-ide	Vasodilators/Nitrates, Cardiovascular	*isosorbide dinitrate* (Isordil), *Isosorbide mononitrate* (Imdur), *nitroprusside* (Nipride)
-ate	Calcium Related Drugs, Endocrine	*tiludronate* (Skelid), *alendronate* (Fosamax), *calcium carbonate* (Tums)
-gliptin	Diabetes DPP-4 Inhibitors, Endocrine	*sitagliptin* (Januvia), *alogliptin* (Nesina), *linagliptin* (Tradjenta)
-tide	Diabetes GLP-1 Agonists, Endocrine	*exenatide* (Bydureon), *liraglutide* (Victoza)
-ide	Diabetes Sulfonylureas, Endocrine	*glimepiride* (Amaryl), *glyburide* (DiaBeta), *glipizide* (Glucotrol)
-glitazone	Diabetes Thiazolidinediones, Endocrine	*pioglitazone* (Actos), *rosiglitazone* (Avandia)
-tropin	Growth Hormone, Endocrine	*somatropin* (Genotropin),

Section 1: Pharmacological Prefix and Suffix Tables

-ase	Enzymes, Endocrine	*pancrelipase* (Creon), *laronidase* (Aldurazyme), *imiglucerase* (Cerezyme)
-dine	H2 Blockers, Gastrointestinal	*nizatidine* (Axid), *famotidine* (Pepcid), *cemetidine* (Tagamet), *ranitidine* (Zantac)
-zine	Antipsychotics, Psychiatry	*prochlorperazine maleate* (Compazine), *thioridazine* (Mellaril)
-done	Antipsychotics, Psychiatry	*risperidone* (Risperdal), *ziprasidone* (Geodon)
-pramine	Tricyclic Antidepressants, Psychiatry	*trimipramine* (Surmontil), *imipramine* (Tofranil), *amitriptyline* (Elavil)
-mab	TNF Inhibitors, Rhematologic	*adalimumab* (Humira), *infliximab* (Remicade), *certolizumab pegol* (Cimzia)
-parin	Anticoagulants	*heparin, dalteparin* (Fragmin), *fondaparinux* (Arixtra)

HIERARCHY OF MAJOR PHARMACOLOGICAL CLASSES

This section lists an outline of the major drug classes and families. The outline includes a common or "gold standard" medication that can be easily referenced for more in depth study of that class. These medications are used across nursing units and would likely be given in the first years of nursing or used in questions on the NCLEX.

The way the outline is displayed helps one understand the hierarchy and associations of various classes as well as the intended use of the drugs. The purpose of this outline is to give the reader a "bird's eye view".

When applicable, both the generic and trade name of a drug is referenced as such *generic name* (Trade name). Please be aware that a generic medicine can have multiple trade names. This is not meant to be an all-inclusive list. It is also not intended to highlight or market for any particular trade name.

IMMUNE SYSTEM

These pharmaceuticals are grouped because of their function - they all impact the immune system. They include active anti-infective agents such as antibiotics, anti-fungals, anti-virals, anti worm agents, tuberculosis or anti-malarial agents. These types of drugs all actively fight off infection or immune system compromise. In addition, this group includes allergy/cold medicines which counteract the initial response of the immune system to an infection.

Immunologics typically convey passive immunity to a person with an auto-immune disorder. Vaccines stimulate the body's immune system to attack and kill particular disease-causing microorganisims. Obviously, this hierarchy of drugs is important to health and well-being of a diverse range of patients.

1. Anti-infective agents

   a. Anti-bacterials

      i Penicillins: e.g. *amoxicillin* (Amoxil)

      ii Cephalosporins

         1. 1st generation: e.g. *cefazolin* (Ancef)

         2. 2nd generation: e.g. *cefprozil* (Cefzil)

         3. 3rd generation: e.g. *cefdinir* (Omnicef)

         4. 4th generation: e.g. *cefepime* (Maxipime)

      i. Aminoglycosides: e.g. *amikacin* (Amikin)

      ii. Macrolides: e.g. *azithromycin* (Zithromax)

      iii. Quinolones: e.g. *ciprofloxacin* (Cipro)

      iv. Sulfonamides: e.g. *cotrimoxazole* (trimethoprim/sulfamethoxazole)

      v. Tetracyclines: e.g. *doxycycline*

      vi. Carbapenems: e.g. *ertapenem* (Invanz)

      vii. Nitrofuran: e.g. *nitrofurantoin*

      viii. Tricyclic glycopeptide: e.g. *vancomycin*

   b. Anti-fungals

      i. Azoles: e.g. *fluconazole* (Diflucan)

      ii. Echinocandins: e.g. *anidulafungin* (Eraxis)

      iii. Other: *amphotericin B*

    c. Anti-virals

        i. CMV retinitis: e.g. *foscarnet* (Foscavir)

        ii. Hepatitis B/C: e.g. *ribavirin*

        iii. Herpes: e.g. *acyclovir* (Zovirax)

        iv. HIV/AIDS: e.g. *zidovudine* (Retrovir, AZT)

        v. Influenza: e.g. *oseltamivir* (Tamiflu)

        vi. RSV: e.g. *palivizumab* (Synagis)

    d. Anti-parasites: e.g. *metronidazole* (Flagyl)

    e. TB: e.g. *isoniazid/rifampin* (Rifamate)

    f. Anthelmintics/Worms: e.g. *mebendazole* (Vermox)

    g. Anti-malarial agents: e.g. *hydroxychloroquine* (Plaquenil)

2. Allergy/Cold Medicines

    a. Antihistamines: e.g. *diphenhydramine* (Benadryl)

    b. Decongestants: e.g. *mometasone* (Nasonex)

    c. Antitussives: e.g. *benzonatate*

    d. Expectorant: e.g. *guaifenesin* (Mucinex)

3. Immunologics

    a. Immune Globulins: e.g. *IVIG*

    b. Immunomodulators: e.g. *6MP* or *mercaptopurine*

    c. Immunosuppressive agents: e.g. *adlimumab* (Humira)

    d. Interferons: e.g. *Interferon Beta-1b* (Betaseron)

4. Vaccinations: e.g. influenza vaccine

ANATOMIC

Another way to order and study pharmaceuticals is by anatomy and where the drug functions within the body. The following medicines are grouped by a class of anatomical functionality such as neurology, cardiology and so forth.

1. Neurology

    a. Seizure

        i. Barbiturates: e.g. *phenobarbital* (Luminal)

        ii. Benzodiazepines: e.g. *clonazepam* (Klonopin)

        iii. Hydantoins: e.g. *phenytoin* (Dilantin)

        iv. Succinimides: e.g. *ethosuximide* (Zarontin)

        v. Calcium-channel subunit alpha2delta ligands: e.g. *gabapentin* (Neurontin)

        vi. Miscellaneous: e.g. *acetazolamide* (Diamox)

    b. Migraines

        i. Ergotamine derivatives: e.g. *ergotamine* (Ergostat)

        ii. Serotonin 5-HT1 Receptor Agonists: e.g. *rizatriptan* (Maxalt)

        iii. Beta-Blockers: e.g. *propranolol*

        iv. Other: e.g. *valproic acid*

    c. Parkinson's

        i. Anticholinergics: e.g. *benztropine* (Cogentin)

      ii. COMT inhibitors: e.g. *tolcapone* (Tasmar)

      iii. Dopaminergics: e.g. *levodopa*

   d. Alzheimer's: e.g. *donepezil* (Aricept)

   e. Other neurodegenerative diseases: e.g. *nataliizumab* (Tysabri)

2. Eye

   a. Antibiotics: e.g. *gentamicin*

   b. Antivirals: e.g. *trifluridine* (Viroptic)

   c. Other: e.g. *Silver Nitrate*

   d. Antiglaucoma: e.g. *acetazolamide* (Diamox)

   e. Cycloplegic/Mydriatic: e.g. *phenylephrine* (Neo-synephrine)

   f. Eye Steroids: e.g. *dexamethasone* (Decadron)

   g. Eye Antihistamines: e.g. *olopatadine* (Pataday)

   h. Eye non-steroidal anti-inflammatories (NSAIDs) : e.g. *ketorolac* (Acular)

   i. Miotics: e.g. *acetylcholine*

   j. Macular Degeneration: e.g. *pegaptanib* (Macugen)

3. Ear

   a. carbamide peroxide (Debrox)

   b.ciprofloxacin/dexamethasone (Ciprodex)

4. Cardiovascular

   a. Nitrates: e.g. *nitrogylcerin*

   b. Thrombolytics: e.g.*alteplase* (TPA, Activase)

c. Volume expanders: e.g. *albumin* (Albuminar)

d. Inotropes and Pressors

    i. Sympathomimetics: e.g.*dopamine* (Intropin)

    ii. Others: e.g. *digoxin* (Lanoxin)

e. Lipid-lower agents

    i. HMG-CoA reductase inhibitors ("statins") : e.g. *atorvastatin* (Lipitor)

    ii. Statin combinations: e.g. *amlodipine/ atorvastatin* (Caduet)

    iii. Fibric acid derivatives: e.g. *gemfibrozil* (Lopid)

    iv. Bile Acid sequestrants: e.g. *colesevelam* (Welchol)

    v. Others: e.g. *ezetimibe* (Zetia)

f. Hypertension

    i. Hypertensive emergencies: e.g. *nitroprusside sodium*

    ii. ACE inhibitors

        1. Angiotension-converting enzyme (ACE) inhibitors: e.g. *benazepril* (Lotensin)

        2. ACE inhibitor/Ca-channel blocker combinations: e.g. *benazepril/amlodipine* (Lotrel)

        3. ACE inhibitor/diuretic combinations: e.g. *enalapril/HCTZ*

    i. Angiotensin II receptor blockers: e.g. *losartan* (Cozaar)

    ii. ARB/diuretic combinations: e.g. *losartan/ HCTZ* (Hyzaar)

    iii. ARB/Ca-channel blocker combinations: e.g. *amlodipine/valsartan* (Exforge)

g. Renin inhibitor: e.g. *aliskiren* (Tekturna)

h. Alpha blockers

    i. Selective alpha-1 adrenergic blockers: e.g. *doxazosin* (Cardura)

    ii. Nonselective alpha adrenergic blockers: e.g. *phentolamine* (Regitine)

i. Beta blockers

    i. Without intrinsic sympathomimetic activity: e.g. *atenolol* (Tenormin)

    ii. With intrinsic sympathomimetic activity: e.g. *penbutolol* (Levatol)

    iii. Combined alpha and beta blockers : e.g. *carvedilol* (Coreg)

    iv. Combined beta blocker and potassium channel blocker: e.g. *sotalol* (Betapace)

j. Calcium channel blockers

    i. Nondihydroopyridines: e.g. *verapamil* (Catan)

    ii. Dihydropyridines: e.g. *amlodipine* (Norvasc)

k. Centrally acting antihypertensives: e.g. *clonidine*

l. Vasodilators: e.g. *hydralazine* (Apresoline)

m. Diuretics

    i. Potassium sparing: e.g. *spironolactone* (Aldactone)

    ii. Thiazides: e.g. *hydrochlorothiazide*

    ii. Loop: e.g. *furosemide* (Lasix)

n. Others

    i. Endothelian receptor blockers eg: *ambrisentan* (Letaris)

    ii. *Sildenafil* (Viagra)

o. Antidysrhythmics

    i. Class 1a: e.g. *disopyramide* (Norpace)

    ii. Class 1b: e.g. *lidocaine* (Xylocaine)

    iii. Class 1c: e.g. *flecainide* (Tambocor)

    iv. Class 2: e.g. *propanolol*

    v. Class 3: e.g. *amiodarone* (Pacerone)

    vi. Class 4: e.g. *verapamil*

    vii. Other: e.g. *magnesium sulfate*

5. Pulmonary

a. Asthma/COPD

    i. Beta-adrenergics: e.g. *albuterol*

    ii. Beta-adrenergic combinations: e.g. *fluticasone/salmeterol* (Advair)

iii. Inhaled corticosteroids: e.g. *budesonide* (Pulmicort)

iv. Leukotriene modifiers: e.g. *montelukast* (Singulair)

v. Monoclonal antibodies: e.g. *omalizumab* (Xolair)

vi. Other: e.g. *ipratropium* (Atrovent)

b. Croup: e.g. *racemic epinephrine*

c. Lung surfactants: e.g. *beractant* (Survanta)

d. Oxygen

6. Gastrointestinal

a. Antacids: e.g. *aluminum hydroxide/magnesium hydroxide* (Maalox)

b. Histamine H2 Antagonists: e.g. *famotidine* (Pepcid)

c. Prostaglandins: e.g. *misoprostol* (Cytotec)

d. Proton Pump Inhibitors: e.g. *pantoprazole* (Protonix)

e. Antiflatulents: e.g. *simethicone* (Mylicon)

f. Prokinetic agents: e.g. *metoclopramide* (Reglan)

g. Anticholinergics/Antispasmodics: e.g. *dicyclomine* (Bentyl)

h. Saline laxatives: e.g. *magnesium citrate*

i. Stimulant laxatives: e.g. *senna*

j. Bulk-producing laxatives: e.g. *psyllium*

k. Emollient laxatives: e.g. *mineral oil* (Milkinol)

l. Stool softeners: e.g. *docusate sodium* (Colace)

m. Bowel evacuant: e.g. *polyethylene glycol* (Miralax)

n. Antidiarrheals: e.g. *loperamide* (Immodium)

o. Antiemetics: e.g. *promethazine* (Phenergan)

p. Diet/weight loss drugs: e.g. *orlistat* (Xenical)

7. Dermatology

a. Antibacterials: e.g. *mupirocin* (Bactroban)

b. Antifungals: e.g. *amphotericin B topical* (Fugizone)

c. Antilice/Scabies: e.g. lindane (Kwell)

d. Topical steroids: e.g. *hydrocortisone*

e. Acne: e.g. *isotretinoin* (Accutane)

f. Wound care: e.g. *collagenase* (Santyl)

g. Other: e.g. *acyclovir topical* (Zovirax)

SYSTEMIC PHARMACEUTICALS

The following drugs act systemically throughout the body to produce intended effects. These include anesthetics, palliative drugs, hematology/oncology, psychiatric medicines, and vitamins.

1. Anesthesia

a. Induction agents: e.g. *thiopental* (Pentothal)

b. Premedication: e.g. *glycopyrrolate* (Robinul)

    c. General anesthetics: e.g. *propofol* (Diprivan)

    d. Neuromuscular blockers: e.g. *vecuronium* (Norcuron)

2. Pain Management

    a. NSAIDS

        i. Acetic Acids

        ii. Fenamates

        iii. Napthylakanones

        vi. Oxicams

        v. Proprionic acids

        vi. Pyranocaboxylic acids

        vii. Pyrrolizine carboxylic acids

        viii. Salicylates

        ix. Selective COX-2 inhibitors

        x. Pyrazolone derivative

    b. Narcotics

        i. Phenanthrenes: Agonists: e.g. *hydromorphone* (Dilaudid)

        ii. Synthetic agonists

            1. Phenylpiperidines: e.g. *fentanyl* (Sublimaze)

            2. Diphenylheptanes: e.g. *propoxyphene* (Darvon)

            3. Other: e.g. *tramadol* (Ultram)

   iii. Partial Agonists: e.g. *nalbuphine* (Nubain)

  c. Muscle relaxants: e.g. *cyclobenzaprine*

  d. Other: e.g. *acetaminophen* (Tylenol)

  e. Local anesthetics

   i. Amides: e.g. *lidocaine*

   ii. Esters: e.g. *procaine* (Novacain)

3. Metabolic/Endocrine

  a. Diabetes

   i. Sulfonylureas: e.g. *glimepiride* (Amaryl)

   ii. Alpha-glucosidase inhibitors: e.g. *miglitol* (Glyset)

   iii. Biguanide: e.g. *metformin*

   iv. DPP-4 Inhibitors: e.g. *sitagliptin*

   v. Hormones: e.g.

    1. *glucagon*

    2. insulin

   vi. Meglitinides: e.g. *nateglinide* (Starlix)

   vii. Thiazolidinediones: e.g. *rosiglitazone* (Avandia)

  b. Thyroid: e.g. *levothyroxine* (Synthroid)

  c. Corticosteroids: e.g. *methylprednisolone* (Solu-medrol)

  d. Sex steroids/Androgens

   i. Anabolic steroids: e.g. *oxymetholone* (Anadrol)

ii. Androgens: e.g. *fluoxymesterone* (Halotestin)

iii. Estrogen - Contraceptives: e.g. *levonorgestrel* (Mirena)

iv. Estrogens: e.g. *estradiol*

v. Progestins: e.g. *medroxyprogesterone* (Provera, depo-provera)

e. Infertility Drugs: e.g. *urofollitropin* (Bravelle)

f. Gout: e.g. *allopurinol*

g. Inborn errors of metabolism: e.g. *agalsidase alfa* (Replagal)

h. Phosphate scavengers: e.g. *sevelamer* (Renagel)

i. Potassium metabolism modifier: e.g. *sodium polystyrene sulfonate* (Kayexalate)

j. Hyperprolactinemia: e.g. *cabergoline* (Dostinex)

k. Acidifying & alkalinizing agents: e.g. *potassium citrate* (Urocit-K)

l. Adrenal function: e.g. *cosyntropin* (Cortosyn, ACTH)

m. Vasopressin-related: e.g. *desmopressin* (DDAVP)

n. Calcium metabolism modifiers

i. Bisphosphonates: e.g. *alendronate* (Fosamax)

ii. Parathyroid function: e.g. *teriparatide* (Forteo)

o. Growth Hormone Related: e.g. *pegvisomant* (Somavert)

4. Hematology

   a. Anticoagulants: e.g. *warfarin* (Coumadin)

   b. Antiplatelet agents: e.g. *clopidrogel* (Plavix)

   c. Hematopoietic growth factors: e.g. *darbepoetin alfa* (Aranesp)

   d. Hemostatics: e.g. *phytonadione* (Vitamin K)

   e. Hemorheologic agents: e.g. *pentoxifylline* (Trental)

   f. Iron Products: e.g. *ferrous sulfate*

   g. Sclerosing agents: e.g. *ethanolamine oleate*

5. Oncology

   a. Alkylating agents: e.g. *cyclophosphamide* (Cytoxan)

   b. Antimetabolites: e.g. *gemcitabine* (Gemzar)

   c. Antimitotic agents: e.g. *cabazitaxel* (Jevtana)

   d. Cytoprotective agents: e.g. *amifostine* (Ethyol)

6. Psychiatry

   a. Benzodiazepines

      i. Short-acting: e.g. *alprazolam* (Xanax)

      ii. Intermediate-acting: e.g. *lorazepam* (Ativan)

      iii. Long-acting: e.g. *clonazepam* (Klonopin)

   b. Benzodiazepine receptor agonists: e.g. *zolpidem* (Ambien)

   c. Barbiturates: e.g. *butabarbital* (Butisol)

   d. Nonbenzodiazepine-nonbarbiturates

      i. Anxiolytic: e.g. *buspirone* (BuSpar)

      ii. Hypnotic: e.g. *doxylamine* (Unisom)

  e. Antidepressants

      i. Selective serotonin reuptake inhibitors: e.g. *citalopram* (Celexa)

      ii. Serotonin norepinephrine reuptake inhibitors: e.g. *duloxetine* (Cymbalta)

      iii. Selective norepinephrine reuptake inhibitor: e.g. *reboxetine* (Vestra)

      iv. Tricyclic antidepressants (TCAs)

         1. Secondary amines: e.g. *amoxapine* (Asendin)

         2. Tertiary amines: e.g. *amitriptyline* (Elavil)

      v. MAO inhibitors: e.g. *phenelzine* (Nardil)

      iv. Other: e.g. *buproprion* (Wellbutrin)

  e. Antipsychotic drugs

      i. Conventional (Typical) agents: e.g. *haloperidol* (Haldol)

      ii. Atypical antipsychotics: e.g. *risperidone* (Risperdal)

  f. Addiction treatment

      i. Alcoholism: e.g. *disulfiram* (antabuse)

      ii. Smoking cessation: e.g. *nicotine*

iii. Stimulants: e.g. *dexmethylphenidate* (Focalin)

7. Vitamins & Minerals

a. Fat-soluble vitamins: e.g. Vitamin A: *retinol*

b. Water-soluble vitamins: e.g. Vitamin B12: *cyanocobalamin*

c. Major minerals: e.g. *magnesium chloride*

e. Trace elements: e.g. *iron*

PREGNANCY SPECIFICS

There are specific cautions and categories to acknowledge in pregnancy. Drugs can be classified in categories of varying risk to a developing fetus of A through X. The following are categories published by the FDA and included on all pharmaceutical profiles (CHEMM, 2013).

Pregnancy Categories

- A: Generally acceptable. Controlled studies in pregnant women show no evidence of fetal risk.

- B: May be acceptable. Either animal studies show no risk, but human studies not available or animal studies showed minor risks and human studies done and showed no risk.

- C: Use with caution if benefits outweigh risks. Animal studies show risk and human studies not available or neither animal nor human studies done.

- D: Use in LIFE-THREATENING emergencies when no safer drug available. There is positive evidence of human fetal risk.

- X: Do not use in pregnancy. Risks involved outweigh potential benefits. Safer alternatives exist.

- NA: Information not available.

Pregnancy specific drugs: e.g. *oxytocin* (Pitocin)

CONTROLLED SUBSTANCES:

Controlled substances are narcotic and non-narcotic drugs regulated by the United States Controlled Substances Act. They are placed on Schedules 1-5 based on regulatory definition of abuse potential, medical use, and possible dependence. These are only able to be prescribed by healthcare providers with a federal DEA number. States vary in regulation as to who can apply for a DEA number. Currently nurse practitioners in Florida cannot have DEA numbers, however a nurse practitioner in Georgia is able to have and prescribe with a DEA.

Controlled substance lists are dynamic and are published annually based off of new regulations. Some controlled substances were listed in the above hierarchy, however, here is an explanation of each schedule.

- Schedule I: Substances in this schedule have no currently accepted medical use in the US, a lack of safety, and a high potential for abuse. They may be prescribed in research to be studied. e.g. heroin, or lysergic acid diethylamide (LSD).

- Schedule II: This schedule has a high potential for abuse and dependence. e.g. morphine, codeine, methylphenidate (Ritalin).

- Schedule III: This schedule has a lower potential for abuse and dependence than Schedule II. Examples include: <15mg of hydrocodone (Vicodin), <90 mg of codeine (Tylenol with Codeine), and anabolic steroids.

- Schedule IV: This schedule has a lower potential for abuse than Schedule III. Examples include temazepam (Restoril) and lorazepam (Ativan).

- Schedule V: These have the lowest potential for abuse of controlled substances. Examples include cough preparations with <200mg of codeine/100ml or 100 grams (Robitussin AC) or diphenoxylate hydrochloride and atropine (Lomotil)

NCLEX Style Questions and Rationales

This section includes NCLEX style questions and rationales on the drugs found in Section 1. There is one question included for each row of the table. This provides good practice for many of the families to be found on the NCLEX. Some of the questions focus on the prefix or suffix and perhaps how it may be confused with other names. Other questions focus on a key point to know about that family. Even if the question talks about only one drug in the row; that concept is almost always applicable to any drug with that prefix/suffix, a couple of which are featured in that row. This allows you to learn a key point about that root family and apply it to any drug you see with that root.

QUESTIONS

Cefa-, cepha-	Cephalosporin, Anti-infective	*cefazolin* (Ancef), *cefoxitin* (Mefoxin), *ceftriaxone* (Rocephin), *cephalexin* (Keflex)

1. A 23 year old woman was hospitalized with community acquired pneumonia and a course of cefazolin 500mg IV every eight hours was ordered. She is not allergic to penicillins. Other medications she takes at home include a multivitamin, albuterol as needed, and Yaz. Medication teaching should include the following:

A. To report any signs of hearing loss

B. That this medication has had an effect of liver failure

C. That her contraception coverage may be reduced while taking this medication

D. That constipation may be a side effect

Pre-, Pred-	Steroids	*prednisone* (Sterapred), *prednisolone* (Orapedr)

2. One of your gastrointestinal patients is leaving the office with a six week taper of prednisone as they currently have a Crohn's Disease flare. You should educate them not to stop the prednisone suddenly because -

A. Prednisone induces the body to stop producing natural steroids and they may go into a crisis.

B. Their flare will return.

C. They might start bleeding.

D. They need the entire dose of antibiotics to get better.

Sulfa-	Anti-infective, Sulfonamides	*sulfadiazine, trimethoprim/ sulfamethoxazole* (Bactrim)

3. A 22 year old female patient presents to the emergency room with complaints of fatigue, low-grade fever, and oral ulcers. During her medication reconciliation, she reports recently being prescribed trimethoprim/sulfamethoxazole (Bactrim) and being around a college campus during the flu season. Part of your nursing judgment includes the following:

A. The symptoms are likely unrelated to her medications and is a new disease process.

B. You triage her with normal vitals and recommend that she go to her primary care physician tomorrow as there is a long wait to get back to be evaluated.

C. The symptoms might be a side effect of her medication known as Stevens Johnson Syndrome.

D. Giving her a mask to wear while she is in the waiting room.

Mor-, -mor-	Opioids	*hydromorphone* (Dilaudid), *morphine sulfate* (MS Contin)

4. You are assessing your patients after a shift change, one of which is hospitalized for sickle cell crisis and has been receiving hydromorphone (Dilaudid) 2mg every 4 hours. The primary team has written for that to be discontinued and replaced with morphine sulfate (MS Contin) 10mg every 4 hours. You decide the following:

A. The dose is appropriate as it is equianalgesic to the 2mg of hydromorphone (Dilaudid).

B. You call the attending physician on call to report an excessive dose of narcotics.

C. You give half the dose and check in on the patient frequently to see how they are doing. If they are okay, you will give the other half of the dose.

D. You hold the dose until further clarification.

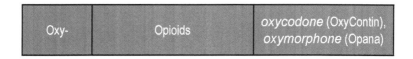

Oxy-	Opioids	*oxycodone* (OxyContin), *oxymorphone* (Opana)

5. A hemodialysis patient on your unit was given 160mg of extended release oxycodone (OxyContin) and is now experiencing vital signs of 80/60, respiratory rate of 8, heart rate of 55, pulse oximetry of 98% and temperature of 98 degrees F. The other

nurse calls you in to help with the patient. After calling a rapid response, you anticipate administering which medication.

A. A saline bolus of 1L IV as quickly as possible.

B. Naltrexone 10mg IV once now

C. Naloxone 2mg IV once now

D. Epinephrine 2mg IV once now

Chole-, cole-	Bile Acid Sequestrants, Cardiovascular	cholestyramine (Questran), colesevelam (Welchol)

6. A patient who is prescribed colesevelam (Welchol) would be correct if they also reported the following lifestyle modifications in order to help the medication's effectiveness.

A. Drinking prune juice daily to counteract constipation

B. Eating an Atkin's type diet to lose weight

C. Monitoring their blood glucose routinely

D. Eating a low-fat, low-cholesterol heart healthy diet

Est-	Estrogens, Endocrine	estradiol vaginal (Premarin), estrogens esterified (Estratest)

7. A 49 year old post-menopausal woman who was previously prescribed estradiol vaginal (Premarin) calls your nurse line to ask whether or not she should take it after having a minor myocardial infarction. Your reply is the following:

A. Yes, it is fine to continue to take.

B. No, it is contraindicated with cardiovascular disease.

C. Yes, it is fine to take since she did not have a stroke.

D. No, she should not take it as she is post-menopausal.

Progest-	Progestins, Endocrine	*progesterone* (Crinone), *medoxyprogesterone* (Provera)

8. A 34 year old woman who smokes and is prescribed medoxyprogesterone (Provera) confides in you that she thinks she might be pregnant. Your next action is to:

A. Give the medication as prescribed

B. Hold the medication until a negative pregnancy test is obtained

C. Recommend that she stop smoking if she is trying to conceive

D. Hold the medication and report to the prescriber that she is a smoker

Cort-	Endocrine, Corticosteroids	*cortisone, hydrocortisone* (Cortef)

9. You are discharging a 3 year old boy with topical hydrocortisone to be applied to his severe eczema. He is allergic to penicillin and also has asthma. The mother conveys her understanding of proper treatment when she says which statement.

> A. I am to apply it once a day to red anywhere on his body
>
> B. I am to apply it twice a day to redness anywhere on his body
>
> C. I am to avoid the genital area and his face when applying the cream
>
> D. I am to apply it every day until he is better.

Tretin-	Dermatology, Anti-cancerous	*tretinoin topical* (Retin-A), *isotretinoin* (Absortica), *Tretinoin ingested* (Vesanoid)

10. A 22 year old woman is being prescribed isotretinoin (Absorica) by her dermatologist. It is most important that she is counseled to take what precautions when taking this pharmaceutical.

> A. Avoid alcohol
>
> B. Wear sunscreen

C. Clean her skin daily before applying

D. Abstain from sex or use two forms of birth control

-sone	Steroids Hormones, Endocrine	prednisone, dexamethasone (Decadron), hydrocortisone (Cortef), fluticasone (Flovent)

11. A 55 year old, African American female is an inpatient on your unit for bacterial meningitis. She has a history of a myocardial infarction, type 2 diabetes mellitus, obesity, and breast cancer. She is receiving dexamethasone (Decadron) for her acute illness. Her vital signs are stable, but her blood glucose level is 310. She says it is normally controlled <150 at home and is concerned about her diabetes. You tell her...

A. Blood glucoses are always higher when you are ill. It will probably come down when you leave the hospital.

B. Let me check your diet and make sure you are receiving a diabetic tray.

C. The illness and steroids you are on are increasing the blood glucose. As you get better, it will return to what it usually is.

D. Maybe your home glucose monitor is not calibrated right. We should check it.

-lone	Steroid Hormones, Endocrine	*prednisolone* (Flo-Pred), *methylprednisolone acetate* (Depo-Medrol), *triamcinolone acetonide* (Trivaris)

12. You notice that your 30 year old juvenile idiopathic arthritis (JIA) female patient who is on long term methylprednisolone is starting to experience a rounded face, thin skin, wasted extremities, and truncal obesity. These are most likely signs of what diagnosis?

A. Obesity

B. Arthritis

C. C Disease

D. Cushing Syndrome

-profen	NSAIDS, Anti-inflammatory	*ibuprofen* (Advil), *flurbiprofen* (Ansaid)

13. You are going to discharge a patient who was admitted to the hospital with abdominal pain and diagnosed on admission with an acute gastrointestinal bleed / ulcers on endoscopy. The team is starting him on omeprazole (Prilosec 40mg PO daily). He frequently takes acetaminophen, naproxen, or ibuprofen for arthritis and migraines.

It is important when you do discharge teaching to advise him to:

  A. Not take any pain medications for at least six weeks.

  B. It is okay to take acetaminophen and naproxen but not ibuprofen.

  C. It is okay to take acetaminophen but not naproxen or ibuprofen.

  D. It is okay for him to take all the medications he is currently on.

-cillin	Penicillin, Anti-infectives	*amoxicillin* (Amoxil), *penicillin, ampicillin/sulbactam* (Unasyn), *piperacillin/tazobactam* (Zosyn)

14. You are caring for a 52 year old woman with a penicillin allergy. She reports that when exposed to the drug she suffers shortness of breath and facial swelling. She has been diagnosed with community-acquired pneumonia. If she were prescribed which drug would you want to hold administration until clarifying with the ordering provider.

  A. Vancomycin (Vancocin) 250mg IV Q 8 hours for 10 days

  B. Ceftaroline (Teflaro) 650mg IV Q 12 hours for 5 days

C. Azithromycin (Z pack) 500mg day 1 then 250mg for 4 days by mouth

D. Amoxicillin clavulanate (Zosyn) 200mg/125mg by mouth Q 12 hours for 10 days

-cycline	Tetracyclines, Anti-infectives	minocycline (Minocin), tetracycline (Sumycin), doxycyclin (Vibramycin)

15. A 22 year old woman presents to the emergency room with acute abdominal and lower back pain. Her last menstrual cycle was 7 weeks ago. She has a history of acne and asthma for which she takes tetracycline and albuterol as needed. You triage her and start screening her for the following:

A. Appendicitis

B. Gastroenteritis

C. Spontaneous abortion (miscarriage)

D. Intimate partner violence

-caine	Anesthetic	prilocaine, marcaine, lidocaine

16. A 55 year old male patient you are taking care of has shingles. The team has prescribed topical lidocaine patches for him to help relieve some of the pain. As you are doing your morning assessment and going to apply new patches, you realize that the night

nurse forgot to remove them. Your patient's vital signs are pain 7/10, 53 heart rate, 10 respirations, 99% oxygen on room air, and 98 F temperature. Appropriate nursing actions would be.

A. Take off the old patches, apply the new patches and reassess pain in 30-60 minutes.

B. Take off the old patches and call a rapid response or code blue.

C. Administer naloxone (Narcan)

D. Take off the old patches and recheck the vital signs in 1 hour.

-nafil	Erectile Dysfunction, Genitourinary, Pulmonary arterial hypertension	*tadalafil* (Cialis), *vardenafil* (Levitra), *sildenafil* (Viagra)

17. A 62 year old male Caucasian patient is admitted to your unit for hypotension at home resulting in syncope. He has a history of hypertension, cataracts, obesity, asthma, and erectile dysfunction. His home medications include hydralazine/hydroclorothiazide 50/50, albuterol HFA 2 puffs every 4-6 hours as needed for wheezing, and sildenafil (Viagra) 25mg as needed. He reports that he is on a low-fat, low-cholesterol diet to help him reduce his weight. He states that a normal blood pressure for him is 140/80 at his doctor's office. Patient education would include the following:

A. Educating him on eating a high fat diet with sildenafil (Viagra) so it works better.

B. Advising him not to take his hydralazine/ hydroclorothiazide 50/5050 with the sildenafil (Viagra).

C. Teaching him to take his blood pressure every day.

D. Teaching him fall precautions.

-prazole	Proton pump inhibitors, Gastrointestional	omeprazole (Prilosec), lansoprazole (Prevacid), esomeprazole (Nexium)

18. Your 30 year old male patient is on omeprazole (Prilosec) 40mg once daily. What dietary teaching is important to give this patient?

A. Avoid citrus, spicy, and tomato-based foods.

B. Take with milk as it will increase absorption.

C. Take the medication 30 minutes after breakfast for best effects.

D. Avoid cream based, high fat foods.

-dipine	Calcium Channel Blockers, Cardiovascular	amlodipine (Norvasc), nifedipine (Adalat), nicardipine (Cardene),

19. Your 38 year old female patient is admitted for pneumonia. She has a history of angina pectoris and breast cancer. She is currently taking nicardipine (Cardene) 20 mg PO daily and piperacillin/ tazobactam (Zosyn) 3.376g IV Q 6 hours. She complains of constipation. The best nursing action would be to do the following:

  A. Increase her oral fluids and encourage her water and fiber intake.

  B. Advocate for her attending to prescribe a stool softener as the constipation is a side-effect of her current medications.

  C. Educate her that if she walks and exercises on the unit more, her constipation will decrease.

  D. Encourage regular toileting routines.

-floxacin	Quinolone, Anti-infectives	*moxifloxacin* (Avelox), *ciprofloxacin* (Cipro), *levofloxacin* (Levaquin)

20. Your 52 year old female patient is suffering from community acquired pneumonia and is an inpatient on a medical surgical floor. She has a history of stroke and asthma. She has no known drug allergies. Her current vital signs are heart rate 79, respiratory rate 21, blood pressure 122/80, temperature 99.0 F, and pulse oximetry 98% on 2L oxygen. Which antibiotic should she not be taking?

A. Moxifloxacin (Avelox) 400mg IV daily

B. Azithromycin (Z pack) 500mg PO daily

C. Vancomycin 500mg IV twice daily

D. Linezolid (Zyvox) 600mg IV BID

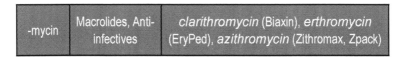

-mycin	Macrolides, Anti-infectives	clarithromycin (Biaxin), erthromycin (EryPed), azithromycin (Zithromax, Zpack)

21. Your 65 year old African American male patient has a history of hypertension, high cholesterol, and obesity. He is allergic to penicillin. He currently takes prevastatin (Prevachol) and amlodipine (Norvasc). He was diagnosed with H. Pylori by your gastroenterology practice and treatment typically includes omeprazole (Prilosec), clarithromycin (Biaxin), and metronidazole (Flagyl). He should take another treatment because -

A. Clarithromycin (Biaxin) is contraindicated in penicillin allergies

B. Those antibiotics will put him at risk for contracting antibiotic resistant strains

C. Prevachol is similar medication as Prilosec so he should not take both at the same time

D. Patients on statins should not take clarithromycin (Biaxin)

-azole	Anti-fungal, Anti-infective Antiparasitic, Anti-infective	*fluconazole* (Diflucan), *itracanazole* (Sporanox), *ketocanazole* *metronidazole* (Flagyl)

22. A 22 year old college sophomore comes into your practice complaining of vaginal irritation and dryness. Her PAP smear tests positive for bacterial vaginosis and she is prescribed metronidazole (Flagyl) 500mg BID for 7 days. Your discharge teaching should include avoiding the following food by mouth while on the medication and for three days afterwards:

A. Grapefruit

B. Dark green leafy vegetables

C. Calcium

D. Alcohol

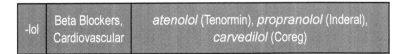

-lol	Beta Blockers, Cardiovascular	*atenolol* (Tenormin), *propranolol* (Inderal), *carvedilol* (Coreg)

23. You are about to discharge a 55 year old man from your medical surgical unit that came in with acute angina. He is going home on carvedilol (Coreg) 100mg twice daily. You decide that your discharge teaching has been effective when he does "teach back" with this high priority learning point:

A. That he should reduce his salt intake in his diet

B. He should not stop taking his medication suddenly

C. He should take an extra dose if he has chest pain

D. He should get daily exercise

-pril	ACE inhibitor, Antihypertensive	*captopril* (Capoten), *lisinopril* (Zestril), *enalapril* (Vasotec)

24. A patient with diabetes type 2 is admitted for several days to your unit. During your review of his home medications, you see that he is supposed to be taking lisinopril (Zestril) 10mg daily. He says that he stopped it because his blood pressure isn't that high and is always around 120/90. Your best response is the following:

A. You tell him that sounds good and strike it from the medical record.

B. You mark the medication as "not being taken at home" and do not say anything to him or his attending.

C. You teach him that ACE inhibitors are often prescribed to decrease the risk and incidence of renal failure in type 2 diabetic patients. You mark the medication as "not being taken at home".

D. You call his doctor immediately.

-sartan	ARB, Antihypertensive	valsartan (Diovan), irbesartan (Avapro), losartan (Cozaar)

25. You have a 33 year old female patient that confides in you during your triage that she is thinking about having a child. Her current medications are the following: ibuprofen (Advil), multi-vitamin, duloxetine (Cymbalta), and valsartan (Diovan). What should you mention she should discuss with her physician or OB-GYN?

    A. Adding a folic acid supplement to her daily medications

    B. Increasing her iron intake

    C. Stopping the duloxetine (Cymbalta)

    D. Stopping the valsartan (Diovan)

-mide, -nide	Loop Diuretics, Cardiovascular	bumeanide (Bumex), furosemide (Lasix), torsemide (Demadex)

26. Which electrolyte is most likely to be decreased in a patient receiving furosemide (Lasix) and what food can replace this electrolyte?

    A. Potassium; Dairy

    B. Magnesium; Milk

    C. Sodium; Sweet potatoes

    D. Calcium; Chicken

-setron	Anti-emetic, Gastrointestional	ondansetron (Zofran), dolasetron (Anzemet)

27. Ondansetron (Zofran) is prescribed to your 47 year old female breast cancer patient. The most probable reason this drug is being given is to:

A. Decrease her appetite

B. Treat cyclic vomiting

C. Treat chemotherapy-induced nausea and vomiting

D. To treat hyperemesis gravidarum

-statin	Anticholesterol Statins, Cardiovascular	lovastatin (Altoprev), rosuvastatin (Crestor), fluvastatin (Lescol)

28. Your 49 year old patient is starting on rosuvastatin (Crestor) 10mg daily. What is a priority teaching in your discharge?

A. To seek immediate medical attention for muscle aches

B. To consider lifestyle changes such as diet and exercise

C. To not stop the medication suddenly

D. To call his doctor if he develops light colored urine

-terol	Bronchodilator/ Beta 2 Agonists	*albuterol sulfate* (Albuterol HFA), *formoterol* (Foradil), *salmeterol* (Serevent)

29. An infant is being discharged from the emergency room on albuterol sulfate to be used every 4 hours as needed for wheezing and cough via a nebulizer. To give this medication, the parents should do the following:

    A. Mix the medicine with an equal part water in the nebulizer cap.

    B. Give the inhaler through a spacer device

    C. Hold the nebulizer tubing up and blow it by the infant's nose

    D. Use a correct size mask on the nebulizer

-thiazide	Thiazide Diuretics, Cardiovascular	chlorothiazide (Diuril), methylclothiazide, hydrochlorothiazide (Microzide)

30. Which electrolyte can be made low and which can be high in a patient that takes hydrochlorothiazide 50mg daily by mouth?

    A. Calcium; Potassium

    B. Potassium; Calcium

    C. Magnesium; Sodium

    D. Sodium; Potassium

-triptan	Anti-migraine, Neurological	*sumatriptan* (Imitrex), *naratriptan* (Amerge), *almotriptan* (Axert)

31. A patient asks you how long he should wait between doses of his sumatriptan while having an acute migraine headache. You tell him the following:

    A. Five minutes

    B. Thirty minutes

    C. Two hours

    D. Four hours

-vir	Antiviral	*ganciclovir* (Cytovene), *valacyclovir* (Valtrex), *acyclovir* (Zovirax), *oseltamivir* (Tamiflu)

32. Your 62 year old patient asks you when they should seek medical attention when taking valacyclovir (Valtrex) for their case of shingles. You tell them the following: *Choose all that apply*

    A. If you do not feel better within 24-48 hours.

    B. If they develop a severe rash.

    C. If they have unexpected red spots on their skin.

    D. If they have a fever or trouble breathing.

-zepam, zolam	Benzodiazepines	*alprazolam* (Xanax), *midazolam* (Versed), *lorazepam* (Ativan), *temazepam* (Restoril), *clonazepam* (Klonopin)

33. Your 30 year old female patient mentions to you that she has been going through a particularly stressful time at work lately and has to take alprazolam (Xanax) throughout the day to help her not have panic attacks at work. What safety concerns is not relevant for this patient.

A. Making sure she understands that if she drives while on this medication, she is under the influence.

B. That she doesn't take more than 2 mg a day.

C. Not to mix alprazolam (Xanax) with alcoholic drinks

D. Not to abruptly stop taking alprazolam (Xanax).

-zosin	Alpha blocker, Cardiovascular	*doxazosin* (Cardura), *terazosin* (Hytrin), *prazosin* (Minipress)

34. Your 58 year old male veteran is taking prazosin (Minipress) 5mg by mouth daily. He is likely taking it for what condition.

A. Benign Prostate Hypertrophy

B. Hypertension

C. Tremors

D. Depression

-cin	Anti-infective, aminoglycosides	*amikacin* (Amikin), *neomycin sulfate*, *tobramycin* (Tobi)

35. Your 18 year old cystic fibrosis patient is being prescribed tobramycin (Tobi) for a respiratory bacterial infection. Before giving it intravenously, you would want to review this black box warning about this medication.

A. It can cause abnormal heart rhythms.

B. If it infiltrates in her vein, it can cause permanent damage to her arm.

C. She should take all doses as prescribed or she might not get better

D. Hearing loss may be irreversible. They should stop the medicine if they experience ringing in their ears or hearing loss and seek medical attention.

-zolamide	Anti-infective, carbonic anhydrase inhibitors	*brinzolamide* (Azopt), *acetazolamide* (Diamox)

36. You are nursing on a medical surgical floor and taking care of a patient with congestive heart failure. The cardiology group has ordered acetazolamide (Diamox) 250mg IV every am to be given to the patient. His vitals are heart rate 77, respiratory rate 18, temperature 98.5F, blood pressure 135/89, and pulse oximetry 98% on room air. He has a history of congestive heart failure and stroke. He is allergic to fish and sulfa. What is your next nursing action?

A. You administer the medication.

B. You hold the medicine and contact the service as that drug is for glaucoma not heart failure.

C. You administer the medication, but monitor the patient's vital signs 30 minutes afterwards

D. You hold the medicine and contact the ordering service as it is contraindicated by his allergy.

-ine	Antihistamines	diphenhydramine (Benadryl), meclizine (Antivert), hydroxyzine (Atarax), loratadine (Claritin), fexofenadine (Allegra),
	Also seen in Antiarrhythmics, Cardiovascular	adenosine (Adenocard), epinephrine (Adrenalin), atropine, dobutamine
	Also seen in immunosuppressants	azathiprine (Azasan), cyclosporine (Gengraf), azathioprine (Imuran)
	Also seen in Antidepressants/SNRIs	duloxetine (Cymbalta), venlafaxine (Effexor)

37. The drug diphenhydramine (Benadryl) makes people sleepy because it exhibits anti-cholinergic effects upon which nervous system of the body.

A. Parasympathetic Nervous System

B. Enteric Nervous System

C. Sympathetic Nervous System

D. Central Nervous System

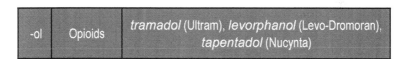

-ol	Opioids	*tramadol* (Ultram), *levorphanol* (Levo-Dromoran), *tapentadol* (Nucynta)

38. A trauma patient is being discharged from your unit with a prescription of tramadol (Ultram) to take for pain at home. She asks if she needs to take any precautions of things not to eat or drink with it. Your best reply is:

A. Grapefruit

B. Alcohol

C. Caffeine

D. Soda

-ium	Neuromuscular Blockers	*vecuronium* (Norcuron), *pancuronium* (Pavulon), *cisatracurium* (Nimbex)

39. Vecuronium (Norcuron) is most given in which unit of the hospital most frequently?

    A. A medical surgical unit

    B. The emergency room

    C. The operating room.

    D. Post anesthesia care unit (PACU)

-penem	Carbapenems, anti-infectives	*ertapenem* (Invanz), *meropenem* (Merem), *doripenem* (Doribax)

40. If a patient is allergic to which substance should they not be given meropenem (Merem)?

    A. Sulfa

    B. Penicillin

    C. Tetracycline

    D. Codeine

-tropium	Anticholinergics, inhaled	*ipratropium bromide* (Atrovent), *tiotropium* (Spiriva)

41. The main purpose of prescribing ipratropium bromide (Atrovent) to a patient is for what action?

A. To bronchodilate the lungs

B. To decrease saliva production

C. To increase diarrhea

D. To increase heart rate

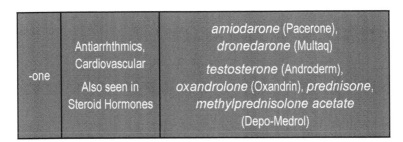

-one	Antiarrhthmics, Cardiovascular Also seen in Steroid Hormones	*amiodarone* (Pacerone), *dronedarone* (Multaq) *testosterone* (Androderm), *oxandrolone* (Oxandrin), *prednisone*, *methylprednisolone acetate* (Depo-Medrol)

42. Your assistant hands you the vital signs for your morning patients. Mr. Smith's vital signs are heart rate 68, respiratory rate 17, temperature 98F, pulse oximetry 98% on 2 L of oxygen, and 80/60 blood pressure. You are about to give him his morning medications which include lansoprazole 30mg, polyethelene glycol 17g, and amiodarone (Pacerone) 800mg. What is your nursing action?

A. Give them all as prescribed

B. Give the lansoprazole and polyethelene glycol but hold the amiodarone and call the attending.

C. Give the lansoprazole but hold the polyethelene glycol and amiodarone and call the attending.

D. Hold them all.

-arin	Anticoagulants, Cardiovascular	*warfarin* (Coumadin), *fondaparinux* (Arixtra), *enoxaparin* (Lovenox)

43. You are taking care of a 55 year old female who was admitted with a thrombus to her left calf. She is being discharged on warfarin (Coumadin) 4 mg daily. What appropriate dietary teaching should you give her?

    A. Do not eat dark green leafy vegetables

    B. Do not eat citrus fruits

    C. Decrease her intake of saturated fats

    D. Decrease sodium in her diet

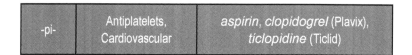

-pi-	Antiplatelets, Cardiovascular	*aspirin, clopidogrel* (Plavix), *ticlopidine* (Ticlid)

44. Your elderly patient was admitted for a fall at home where she bruised her head. X-rays are negative and she is to be discharged with her daughter. Her home medications are the following: one baby aspirin daily, omeprazole 40mg daily, and colace daily. What directions should you give her?

    A. Take all your medications as prescribed.

    B. Do not take any of your medications until your follow up appointment in 2 weeks.

C. Take the colace daily but hold the baby aspirin and omeprazole.

D. Take the colace and the omeprazole but hold the baby aspirin until your doctor restarts it

-plase	Thrombolytics, Cardiovascular	*alteplase* (Activase), *reteplase* (Retavase), *tenecteplase* (TNKase)

45. Alteplase (Activase) is a revolutionary treatment for acute ischemic stroke patients. However, within what timeframe of symptom presentation must it be administered?

A. <2 hours

B. <3 hours

C. <5 hours

D. <10 hours

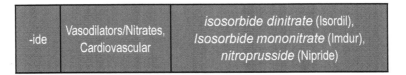

-ide	Vasodilators/Nitrates, Cardiovascular	*isosorbide dinitrate* (Isordil), *Isosorbide mononitrate* (Imdur), *nitroprusside* (Nipride)

46. Your 55 year old patient calls complaining of headache. She just started isosorbide mononitrate (Imdur) today while an inpatient for her frequent chest pain. What is the best thing to tell her?

A. That you can turn off her lights to help.

B. You will try to keep the sound down in the unit.

C. Some as needed pain medication might help

D. That is a very common side effect, keep taking the medicine and it should go away soon.

-ate	Calcium Related Drugs, Endocrine	*tiludronate* (Skelid), *alendronate* (Fosamax), *calcium carbonate* (Tums)

47. Your patient is taking alendronate (Fosamax). What is important to tell them to do after taking the medicine?

A. Eat breakfast

B. Do not lie down or recline for 30 minutes

C. Lie down for 15 minutes

D. Take calcium

-gliptin	Diabetes DPP-4 Inhibitors, Endocrine	*sitagliptin* (Januvia), *alogliptin* (Nesina), *linagliptin* (Tradjenta)

48. Your type 2 diabetic patient is being discharged from the hospital on a new medicine for him sitagliptin (Januvia) along with his previous diabetic medications. As you are reviewing his discharge teaching including the warning signs for his new

medicine, he asks you what abdominal or back pain might indicate. You respond that it is most likely to be associated with the acute onset of:

A. Pancreatitis

B. Gastric ulceration

C. Appendicitis

D. Hypoglycemia

-tide	Diabetes GLP-1 Agonists, Endocrine	*exenatide* (Bydureon or Byetta), *liraglutide* (Victoza)

49. When should exenatide (Byetta) be given to your patient?

A. First thing in the morning

B. Before they go to sleep at night

C. Before each meal and before sleep

D. 1 hour before the meal it is prescribed for

-ide	Diabetes Sulfonylureas, Endocrine	*glimepiride* (Amaryl), *glyburide* (DiaBeta), *glipizide* (Glucotrol)

50. How do sulfonylureas work in the body for diabetics?

A. They are given to type 1 diabetics in order to help them produce more natural insulin

B. They help break down glucose in the food so it doesn't raise blood sugar

C. It is an artificial form of insulin that helps the body process glucose

D. They are given to type 2 diabetics in order to help them produce more natural insulin

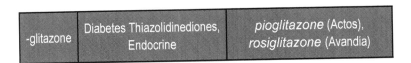

-glitazone	Diabetes Thiazolidinediones, Endocrine	*pioglitazone* (Actos), *rosiglitazone* (Avandia)

51. Glitazones have recently been earmarked with several high risk factors. In particular, rosiglitazone (Avandia) has been shown to be correlated with disorders of which system? It can only be taken if the benefits outweigh the risks and the patient is well-informed.

A. Cardiac

B. Pulmonary

C. Genitourinary

D. Neurological

-ase	Enzymes, Endocrine	*pancrelipase* (Creon), *laronidase* (Aldurazyme), *imiglucerase* (Cerezyme)

52. Your newly diagnosed cystic fibrosis patient's parents ask for directions on taking the pancrelipase (Creon). You tell them she should take it.

   A. Before breakfast

   B. With each meal

   C. Thirty minutes before each meal

   D. Before sleep

-dine	H2 Blockers, Gastrointestinal	*nizatidine* (Axid), *famotidine* (Pepcid), *cemetidine* (Tagamet), *ranitidine* (Zantac)

53. What is the most likely pH of the stomach after a patient takes ranitidine (Zantac)?

   A. 2.0

   B. 1.0

   C. 4.0

   D. 8.0

-zine	Antipsychotics, Psychiatry	*prochlorperazine maleate* (Compazine), *thioridazine* (Mellaril)

54. Your patient is taking prochlorperazine maleate (Compazine) and requests lorazepam for anxiety. Your best response is:

A. To also give the lorazepam

B. To teach that the Compazine will help with the anxiety

C. To call the attending

D. To tell the patient no and go eat your lunch.

-done	Antipsychotics, Psychiatry	risperidone (Risperdal), ziprasidone (Geodon)

55. Risperidone (Risperdal) is typically prescribed for which psychiatric illness?

A. Severe depression

B. Bipolar disorder

C. Anxiety

D. Schizophrenia

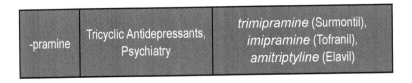

-pramine	Tricyclic Antidepressants, Psychiatry	trimipramine (Surmontil), imipramine (Tofranil), amitriptyline (Elavil)

56. Before starting a patient on amitriptyline (Elavil), it would be important to tell them and document that they know about the black box warning indicating an increased risk of:

A. Heart Attack

B. Stroke

C. Suicide

D. Insomnia

-mab	TNF Inhibitors, Rhematologic	*adalimumab* (Humira), *infliximab* (Remicade), *certolizumab pegol* (Cimzia)

57. Your 18 year old patient is being prescribed infliximab (Remicade) infusions for her inflammatory bowel disease. It is important for her to get which test before starting the infusions.

A. A ppd

B. A dexa scan

C. Another colonoscopy

D. A blood culture

-parin	Anticoagulants	*heparin, dalteparin* (Fragmin), *fondaparinux* (Arixtra)

58. Your 47 year old man is being discharged on heparin injections. What is an important piece of home care teaching to tell him?

A. Massage the site after each injection

B. Do not eat dark green leafy vegetables

C. Only shave with an electric razor with a guard

D. Sleep 8-10 hours a night

Answers and Rationales

1. Correct answer: C - That her contraception coverage may be reduced while taking this medication

Rationale: Cephalosporins commonly have an adverse effect of reducing contraceptive coverage. Percentages vary among research studies. Cephalosporins typically have cefa- or cepha- in the prefix of the generic name of the medication making is easy to generalize this to any medication you see with that prefix.

2. Correct answer: A. Prednisone induces the body to stop producing natural steroids and they may go into a crisis.

Rationale: Prednisone and the steroid hormone family all suppress our natural immune system. When you take a high-dose steroid like prednisone, the body normalizes by decreasing the amount of natural cortisol hormone it produces. If you remove the artificial steroid suddenly, it does not give the body enough time to start making the cortisol to replace it. Your patient can experience an Addison crisis which can be life-threatening if untreated. Their flare might return if they stop the medication and that might also come with bloody stools, but these are not the best answer. Prednisone is not an antibiotic. The steroid family can be recognized by the -sone , -lone, or the pred- stems in the generic name.

3. Correct answer: C - The symptoms might be a side effect of her medication known as Stevens Johnson Syndrome.

Rationale: Stevens Johnson Syndrome is a side effect of infection, medications or disease. It results in flu-like symptoms and ulcers on mucous membranes that can sometimes make it difficult to eat or drink. Left untreated, it can be fatal and result in wide areas of necrosis.

4. Correct answer: A - The dose is appropriate as it is equianalgesic to the 2mg of hydromorphone (Dilaudid).

Rationale: There are many published charts on equianalgesic dosing that you can find in pharmacology references. The ratio essentially is that 2mg hydromorphone: 10mg morphine sulfate. You must read the charts carefully for drug type as well as route. What this means that if you give a patient 2 mg of hydromorphone (Dilaudid) and then their medication is switched to morphine sulfate, then they have to get at least 10mg to have the same analgesic effect. There are actually no published upper limits to pain medication. Pain medication is dosed per a patient's reaction to minimize pain and side effects such as respiratory depression. Some patients that build up a tolerance over time may require very high doses to achieve the same effect.

5. Correct answer: C - Naloxone 2mg IV once now

Rationale: Naloxone (Narcan) is the opioid antagonist of choice when treating opioid induced respiratory depression. It is commonly administered every 2-3 minutes as symptoms necessitate and is typically found in unit code-carts. Note that opioids could have the oxy- or mor- prefix. You would use naloxone to counteract any medication with this prefix.

6. Correct answer: D - Eating a low-fat, low-cholesterol heart healthy diet

Rationale: Colesevalam (Welchol) is commonly prescribed for the purpose of lowering cholesterol. It binds to cholesterol in the GI system, which decreases its absorption thus improving cholesterol levels. It is meant to enhance healthy lifestyle choices such as heart healthy eating and exercise habits. The prefix chole- or cole- is a Greek term that means "relating to bile or the bile ducts". In medications or other terms with this prefix, it will related to bile, cholesterol, gallbladder, or the liver.

7. Correct answer: B - No, it is contraindicated with cardiovascular disease.

Rationale: Estrogens are contraindicated in women with cardiovascular disease, hypothyroidism, diabetes mellitus, hypocalcemia, breast cancer, or DVTs. They have been shown to increase the risk of cardiovascular events including stroke, memory loss, and dementia. Currently the FDA regulates that they carry a Black Box warning to this effect. Generic names with the prefix est- can be recognized as being part of this family, although it is very common to refer to medications in this group by trade names rather than generics. Generally, estrogens can be found in many contraceptives as well as hormones.

8. Correct answer: B - Hold the medication until a negative pregnancy test is obtained

Rationale: While progesterones are cautioned in smokers, it is not completely contraindicated and might be given when risks are outweighed by benefits. However, it is a pregnancy X medication and could have teratogenic effects on a fetus causing fetal demise, spontaneous abortion, or fetal malformation. Medications that are progesterones will have the progest- stem somewhere in their generic name. However, this family of medications is also commonly referred to in the vernacular by their trade names to distinguish them clinically.

9. Correct answer: C - I am to avoid the genital area and his face when applying the cream

Rationale: Hydrocortisone is only to be applied for less than 7 days and in areas that do not include the genitals and the face. These areas have very thin layers of skin that might absorb too much hydrocortisone causing hypopigmentation or atrophy. Any medication with the "cort" stem in the name can be part of the cortisone family and should adhere to this precaution.

10. Correct answer: D. Abstain from sex or use two forms of birth control

Rationale: Isotretinoin (Absorica) is an oral drug taken to help eradicate severe acne. Although it is important to wear sunscreen and have good skin hygiene, the most important nursing counseling is to avoid becoming pregnant. Patients typically have to sign waivers, be educated, and have two pregnancy tests before taking this medication. It is a pregnancy X medication and can cause spontaneous abortion or fetal malformation. This black box warning extends to most oral forms of the tretin family, however does not pertain to the topical formulations.

11. Correct answer: C. The illness and steroids you are on are increasing the blood glucose. As you get better, it will return to what it usually is.

Rationale: Steroids increase the production of glucose (gluconeogenesis) and decrease the utilization of glucose thus resulting in hyperglycemia. Patients with diabetes may need adjustment to their therapy. Nondiabetic patients may develop iatrogenic diabetes during their course of treatment. Acute illness also elevates blood glucose levels. The steroid family can be recognized by the -sone , -lone, or the pred- stems in the generic name.

12. Correct answer: D - Cushing Syndrome

Rationale: Cushing Syndrome can be caused by prolonged exposure to steroids. It is epitomized by rapid weight gain, a moon face, thin skin, easy bruising, and central obesity. Cushing Disease is similar but is caused by a tumor that encroaches on the adrenals or pituitary gland. The steroid family can be recognized by the -sone , -lone, or the pred- stems in the generic name.

13. Correct answer: C - It is okay to take acetaminophen but not naproxen or ibuprofen.

Rationale: Actaminophen (Tylenol) is excreted through the liver and does not have side effects that would increase gastrointestinal bleeding. However, naproxen and ibuprofen are both NSAIDS or non-steroidal anti-inflammatory drugs. A common side effect of all NSAIDS is to increase stomach upset and the risk of GI bleeding.

14. Correct answer: D. Amoxicillin clavulanate (Zosyn) 200mg/125mg by mouth Q 12 hours for 10 days

Rationale: The basic question is what drug should you not give a patient with a penicillin allergy. Although azithromycin and vancomycin both sound like -cillin, they are macrolides and "other" respectively, not penicillins. Teflaro (Ceftaroline) is a distractor because it is a cephalosporin. First - fourth generation cephalosporins are not to be given to patients but since Teflaro is a fifth generation, then it is okay. Amoxicillin clavulnate (Zosyn) is the correct answer. It is a penicillinase and would cause a severe reaction.

15. Correct answer: C. Spontaneous abortion (miscarriage)

Rationale: The tetracycline family is labeled pregnancy D or positive evidence of maternal-fetal risk. It is not to be given to pregnant or lactating women as the risk outweighs the benefits. Although appendicitis, gastroenteritis, and intimate partner violence are all to be considered due to her age, a nurse should screen her for sexual activity and birth control methods as well. Medications within this family can be recognized by their -cycline suffix in many generic names.

16. Correct answer: B. Take off the old patches and call a rapid response or code blue.

Rationale: The -caine family can cause overdose in patients with overdose or prolonged exposure. Signs of overdose include bradycardia, uneven heart rhythms, seizures, slowed breathing, or coma. Topical lidocaine patches are only to be left on for 12 hours. Due to the patient's age, morbidity, warmth, and application of the patches, he may be experiencing overdose. The most important nursing action is to remove the lidocaine and initiate the response team to stabilize the patient. Naloxone (Narcan) is an opioid antagonist and would not have an effect on this anesthetic family. This family can be reversed with lipid emulsions instead.

17. Correct answer: B. Advising him not to take his hydralazine/ hydroclorothiazide 50/5050 with the sildenafil (Viagra).

Rationale: Nitrates such as hydralazine/hydroclorothiazide also cause vasodilation. When taken with sildenafil (Viagra) or other medications in that family, they can cause fatal hypotension. This warning extends to all generic medications with the -nafil suffix. Patients are to avoid taking any nitrates while taking erectile dysfunction medication. Eating a high fat diet actually decreases the effectiveness of sildenafil. Taking his blood pressure daily and having fall precautions should also be done but are not the best answer.

18. Correct answer: A. Avoid citrus, spicy, and tomato-based foods.

Rationale: Medications that are proton pump inhibitors come with the -prazole suffix. They are given to reduce gastric acid in the stomach leading to decreased damage from acid reflux and promoting a healing environment for peptic. Patients taking these medications should avoid highly acidic foods such as citrus or spicy foods that may aggravate their underlying condition. The medication should be taken 30 minutes before breakfast for best absorption.

19. Correct answer: B. Advocate for her attending to prescribe a stool softener as the constipation is a side-effect of her current medications.

Rationale: Calcium channel blockers such as nicardipine (Cardene) inhibit the calcium influx in between cells but specifically to smooth muscle in the gut and heart. The action of reducing afterload on the heart helps in conditions such as angina or hypertension but also decreases contractility of the bowel smooth muscle contributing to constipation. Taking a daily stool softener might help this chronic side-effect. Calcium channel blockers include those with -dipine that are not approved as anti-arrhythmics as well as verapamil (Calan) and diltiazem (Cardizem) that are also approved as anti-arrhythmics.

20. Correct answer: A. Moxifloxacin (Avelox) 400mg IV daily

Rationale: Moxifloxacin (Avelox) is a quinolone. This family is especially known for its black box warning for possible tendon rupture. It also has contraindications to any type of disorder affecting the central nervous system such as a stroke as it can cause psychosis or CNS toxicity. In addition, cardiac patients also must be monitored closely for QT prolongation. Although their name has a -in ending, they are not part of the penicillin family but rather their own root ending with -floxacin.

21. Correct answer: D. Patients on statins should not take clarithromycin (Biaxin)

Rationale: Statins are contraindicated with macrolide use and can lead to myopathy. Macrolides include clarithromycin, erythromycin, azithromycin and other drugs with the root ending of -mycin. Although clarithromycin has a -in ending, it is not a penicillin but a macrolide. Taking multiple antibiotics can cause antibiotic resistance, but clearly the benefits of taking antibiotics as recommended for his H. pylori outweighs the risk. Antibiotic use is generally discouraged when not indicated by practice guidelines. Prevachol sounds like Prevacid, another proton pump inhibitor such as omeprazole (Prilosec) but it is a statin.

22. Correct answer: D. Alcohol

Rationale: Alcohol can react with this anti-infective family of -azoles but giving the patient symptoms of toxicity, nausea, vomiting, and flushing. Grapefruit is to be avoided with many medications as it can dangerously raise drug levels in the blood but flagyl is not one of them. Dark green leafy vegetables contain high amounts of vitamin K and are to be avoided in those patients taking Coumadin. Calcium can interfere with the body's ability to use several other antibiotics such as tetracycline.

23. Correct answer: B. He should not stop taking his medication suddenly

Rationale: Beta blockers such as those ending in the -lol root should not be stopped suddenly. These medications contain a black box warning to that effect because if they are, then the patient might suffer heart attack, severe chest pain, or heart arrhythmias that could be fatal.

24. Correct answer: C. You teach him that ACE inhibitors are often prescribed to decrease the risk and incidence of renal failure in type 2 diabetic patients. You mark the medication as "not being taken at home".

Rationale: ACE inhibitors end in the root -pril. One example is lisinopril (Zestril). Although these are commonly prescribed for hypertension, they also can be prescribed to type 2 diabetics that are at risk for renal damage.

25. Correct answer: D. Stopping the valsartan (Diovan)

Rationale: Valsartan (Diovan) and other ARB antihypertensives that end in -sartan have a black box warning for use in pregnancy. In women trying to get pregnant or women that are pregnant, they should consider switching medications with their prescriber. The other options are all good, but answer D might prevent fetal demise.

26. Correct answer: A. Potassium; Dairy

Rationale: All loop diuretics that end in -mide or -nide such as "furosemide (Lasix)" decrease the capability of the body to recycle potassium. As such, potassium can be decreased and needed by the body. Dairy products, potatoes, beans, apricots, fish, salmon among others are foods high in potassium. Diuretics may also decrease other electrolytes such as magnesium, sodium, and calcium - but the first one to be depleted will be potassium and it is of the greatest concern.

27. Correct answer: C. Treat chemotherapy-induced nausea and vomiting

Rationale: The -setron root depicts medications that act as anti-emetic agents in the central nervous system. They reduce nausea associated with chemotherapy or radiation in oncology patients. They can also be used for other forms of nausea but with this patient's diagnosis, is most likely prescribed for that purpose.

28. Correct answer: A. To seek immediate medical attention for muscle aches

Rationale: Muscle aches are a sign of a condition that might be triggered by taking a statin called rhabdomyolysis where skeletal muscle is dissolved and can cause acute renal failure. Patients with this condition should immediately stop their statin and seek medical attention. Lifestyle changes are important as the primary reason statins are prescribed are for reducing cholesterol. Dark colored urine can be a sign of renal damage and the patient should also call their prescriber.

29. Correct answer: D. Use a correct size mask on the nebulizer

Rationale: Bronchodilators are given through inhaled routes by using inhalers, spacer devices, nebulizers and sometimes metered dose inhalers. The correct position, breathing technique, and use of equipment is very important to receive the dose of medication. This is a very important part of nursing teaching and questioning on intake or discharge. Bronchodilators are typically found with the "-terol" root.

30. Correct answer: B. Potassium; Calcium

Rationale: Hydrochlorothiazides act on the distal tubules of the kidney to reduce sodium absorption causing diuresis. Therefore sodium, magnesium, and potassium can be lower in persons taking this medicine. Its action also increases the uptake of calcium in the kidneys in an unrelated fashion, which can make calcium levels higher than normal.

31. Correct answer: C. Two hours

Rationale: Sumatriptan is part of the triptan family. It narrows blood vessels around the brain, decreasing the inflammation that can contribute to migraines. Taking multiple doses within two hours can cause adverse cardiac or stroke events. With both tablets or nasal sprays, patients should wait two hours and only repeat the dose if the headache is still occurring.

32. Correct answer: B, C, and D.

Rationale: Valacyclovir (Valtrex) is part of a group of drugs known as anti-virals. These typically end in the -vir root. They do not attack the current virus in the body but help prevent it from replicating. Therefore, they can shorten or lessen the severity of an illness but do not eradicate it quickly. Many serious side effects can happen but rarely do. Patients should be informed to seek medical attention for a severe rash called Steven-Johnson's syndrome that can be fatal. Red or purple spots on skin can be symptoms of leukopenia or neutropenia or a hemolytic-uremic syndrome (HUS). HUS can cause destruction of red blood cells leading to acute renal failure and fatality if not treated. Fever and anaphylaxis would also be non-specific signs of reasons to seek immediate medical care.

33. Correct answer: B. That she doesn't take more than 2 mg a day.

Rationale: The maximum dose of alprazolam (Xanax) is typically around 4mg/day. This is a benzodiazepine family medication, which typically end in -zepam or -zolam roots. These medications are considered controlled substances in the United States and it is illegal to obtain them without a prescription. Driving while on this medication, can be a D.U.I. if a driver appears unsafe. Alcohol can increase the affects of benzodiazepines and should not be mixed. Respiratory or central nervous system depression can result. Abruptly stopping a benzodiazepine can lead to withdrawal symptoms that typically result in irritability, jitters, insomnia, or manic-like symptoms.

34. Correct answer: A. Benign Prostate Hypertrophy

Rationale: Alpha blockers can be prescribed for three reasons - typically benign prostate hypertrophy (BPH), hypertension, or anxiety related disorders such as PTSD. When taken for BPH, the dose is low, about 5mg or less. When taking for hypertension, the dose is typically around 15mg. Prescribing for psychiatric concerns is currently in research and is an off-label use that dosages are still being developed for. Alpha blockers can be recognized because they typically end in the root -zosin.

35. Correct answer: D. Hearing loss may be irreversible. They should stop the medicine and seek medical attention if they experience ringing in their ears or hearing loss.

Rationale: Aminoglycosides are well known for their potential side-effects of ototoxicity (ear damage) or nephrotoxicity (kidney damage). As these medications typically end in -cin roots, they can be easy to spot. Although very effective against certain bacterial infections, they can cause irreversible ear damage quickly or weeks after administration. Abnormal heart rhythms and infiltration are not black box warnings on this medication. Black box warnings are specific risks required by the FDA to be on particular medicines.

36. Correct answer: D. You hold the medicine and contact the ordering service as it is contraindicated by his allergy.

Rationale: Pharmaceuticals that end in "-zolamide" are carbonic anhydrase inhibitors. They contain a set of organic molecules called the "sulfonamides" in them. The sulfonamide group forms the base of sulfa drugs and carbonic anhydrase inhibitors. Therefore people that are allergic to sulfa drugs will also be allergic to any drug ending in -zolamide. Diamox is given for several indications including glaucoma, altitude sickness, or congestive heart failure and comes in PO/IV form. Brinzolamide (Azopt) is typically given for glaucoma and comes as eye drops.

37. Correct answer: A. Parasympathetic Nervous System

Rationale: The parasympathetic nervous system (PNS) is the system of the body that controls involuntary movements. Diphenhydramine and other antihistamines act with an anticholinergic effect and block the binding of the neurotransmitter acetylcholine to its receptors in nerve cells.

38. Correct answer: B. Alcohol

Rationale: Tramadol (Ultram) is part of the family of opioids. Opioids naturally depress the body which helps minimize pain. However, if taken with other substances that cause depression in the body such as alcohol, narcotics, or other medications - then they can cause respiratory depression. This can result in death.

39. Correct answer: C. The operating room.

Rationale: Vecuronium (Norcuron) is a neuromuscular blocker as is other medicines ending in -ium such as pancuronium and cisatracurium. They are used for skeletal muscle relaxation during surgery or intubation. Although they may be given in an ICU, they are commonly only given in the operating rooms of the hospital to supplement anesthesia care.

40. Correct answer: B. Penicillin

Rationale: Carbapenems are a large class of beta-lactam antibiotics. They fight against a broad spectrum of bacteria. A carbapenem is actually the 4:5 fused ring lactam of penicillins. Therefore patients that are allergic to penicillin are also allergic to carbapenems. These are easily recognized by the "-penem" root. At this time, most carbapenems are given via intravenous routes.

41. Correct answer: A. To bronchodilate the lungs

Rationale: Ipratropium bromide (Atrovent) and tiotropium (Spiriva) are both anticholinergics. You can recognize them with the "-tropium" ending. They act on the parasympathetic system to block acetylcholine from acting. Therefore, they relax smooth muscle throughout the body. Although ipratropium bromide will decrease saliva production, increase diarrhea, and increase heart rate, its most important function for which it is commonly prescribed is to bronchodilate the lungs. It allows those with COPD or asthma to breathe easier.

42. Correct answer: B. Give the lansoprazole and polyethelene glycol but hold the amiodarone and call the attending.

Rationale: The patient's blood pressure is quite low at 80/60. A common side effect of amiodarone is hypotension. If you were to give the medicine, it may endanger the patient. Holding the medicine and calling the physician on duty immediately is the best course of action at this point. Amiodarone and dronedarone are both anti-arrhythmics. They work on the heart to prolong the action potential.

43. Correct answer: A. Do not eat dark green leafy vegetables

Rationale: Warfarin (Coumadin) helps thin a person's blood so as to prevent the recurrence of thrombus or embolism. The antagonist to warfarin is Vitamin K. Indeed, if a patient is admitted with an INR level that is too high, often a nurse will be ordered to give them shots of Vitamin K. Vitamin K is found naturally in dark, green, leafy vegetables such as collards and spinach. Therefore, patients should avoid eating these as it can quickly decrease their INR level, leading to potential for clots to occur. You can recognize other anticoagulants by their "-arin" root.

44. Correct answer: D. Take the colace and the omeprazole but hold the baby aspirin until your doctor restarts it

Rationale: Aspirin as with other antiplatelets, slows the clotting function of platelets in our blood. This increases the risk of bleeding. Aspirin is contraindicated in persons with recent trauma, ulcers, strokes, as well as certain liver, kidney, or blood disorders. Antiplatelets can be recognized by the small root of "-pi-" within the generic name.

45. Correct answer: B. <3 hours

Rationale: The quote "time is brain" comes to mind. These thrombolytics above, recognized by their -plase root are revolutionizing the ability to treat strokes and preserve neurological function. However, current clinical guidelines state that they should be used within 3 hours of symptom onset and after a CT is obtained to rule out hemorrhage.

46. Correct answer: D. That is a very common side effect, keep taking the medicine and it should go away soon.

Rationale: Isosorbide mononitrate (Imdur) has the action of vasodilating vessels in the body. It is used primarily to prevent angina from occurring. The vasodilation has the consequential effect of increasing blood flow to the brain resulting in headaches when the medication is started. These should go away quickly with continued treatment and only 2-3% of patients have to stop therapy. Distractions and prn medication may help but the most important thing to do is reassure the patient not to stop the medication. Other vasodilators also end in the "-ide" root such as isosorbide dinitrate and nitroprusside.

47. Correct answer: B. Do not lie down or recline for 30 minutes

Rationale: Alendronate (Fosamax) is a medicine called a bisphosphonate drug used to counteract osteoporosis. Intake with food or drinks will inhibit the uptake of the medicine. However, patients should sit upright, stand or walk for 30 minutes after taking the medicine because lying down can contribute to ulcerations of the stomach or esophagus. You can recognize other bisphosphonates due to the -ate root that is in their generic names.

48. Correct answer: A. Pancreatitis

Rationale: Sitagliptin (Januvia) works by regulating the pancreas and the way it releases insulin. There is a risk associated with it of pancreatitis. Pancreatitis can manifest with right upper quadrant abdominal pain or referred back pain. Gastric ulcerations and appendicitis are not at an increased risk with Januvia intake. Hypoglycemia can happen, but would not be associated with pain. The DPP-4 inhibitors all carry this increased risk as they alter the pancreatic functioning. You can easily identify this class of drugs with its -gliptin root.

49. Correct answer: D. 1 hour before the meal it is prescribed for

Rationale: Exenatide (Byetta) is a diabetes GLP-1 agonist. It helps a patient's pancreas work more efficiently. Therefore, it is always scheduled to be given 1 hour before meals. Typically it is prescribed twice a day. This class of medications can be found by the -tide root in the generic name.

50. Correct answer: D. They are given to type 2 diabetics in order to help them produce more natural insulin

Rationale: Sulfideonylureas such as glimeptride (Amaryl) help the pancreatic beta cells produce more insulin. For this reason, they can only be given to new type 2 diabetics. Type 1 diabetics have no functional beta cells. Type 2 diabetics that have been diagnosed for a long period of time, might as well have very few functioning beta cells. This class of medications can be recognized by their -ide ending. It is similar to the -tide ending found in the GLP-1 Agonists family because they do the same function.

51. Correct answer: A. Cardiac

Rationale: The glitazone family works by making cells more responsive to insulin. Rosiglitazone (Avandia) has been shown to be correlated with an increased risk of heart attacks, making it less desirable. Patients have to sign informed consent before receiving it. The glitazone family is easily recognized with its key root ending in generic names.

52. Correct answer: With each meal

Rationale: Medications ending in -ase are part of a class that make up artificial pancreatic enzymes when disorders prevent the body from producing them. Our pancreas ejects enzymes into our digestive tract when we eat to help break down food and absorb nutrients. Thus, the enzymes should be eaten at the start of the meal.

53. Correct answer: C. 4.0

Rationale: Ranitidine as with other H2 blockers decreases acid production in the stomach. In doing so, the pH of the stomach is changed from one that is low (e.g. 2.0) to more basic or a higher pH (4.0). The pH scale goes from 1 to 14 with 7.0 being the dividing line. Ph readings < 7.0 are acidic, while pH readings > 7.0 are basic. This helps prevent ulcerations from occurring. The normal pH of the stomach ranges from 1-3.0. When a dose of a H2 blocker (ranitidine) or proton pump inhibitor (omeprazole) is given, then the pH becomes more basic around 4.0. It does not actually become "basic" as in > 7.0.

54. Correct answer: B. To teach that the Compazine will help with the anxiety

Rationale: This class of medicines are dopamine antagonists. By blocking dopamine's action in the brain, they decrease anxiety, nausea, vomiting, vertigo, and migraines. Giving too much of anything that will also cause respiratory or physical depression may result in demise of the patient. Monitor their vitals closely. This class is quickly spotted by the -zine root.

55. Correct answer: D. Schizophrenia

Rationale: Antipsychotics are typically prescribed for psychiatric illnesses such as schizophrenia. Sometimes they are prescribed as an adjunctive to help with bipolar depression.

They can easily be recognized by their -done root.

56. Correct answer: C. Suicide

Rationale: Most antidepressants, including the tricyclics now carry a black box warning mandated by the FDA that they are associated with an increased risk of suicide. Tricyclic antidepressants can be easily identified with the -pramine root.

57. Correct answer: A. A ppd

Rationale: Taking any of the TNF inhibitors can put the patients at risk for severe pulmonary/fungal diseases including TB. Getting a ppd before starting therapy is part of the clinical guidelines and should be anticipated.

58. Correct answer: C. Only shave with an electric razor with a guard

Rationale: Anticoagulants all work by thinning the blood, creating a high risk of bleeding. Men and women should be told not to use sharp razors to shave after being prescribed heparin. Massaging the site might do underlying tissue damage. This class is easily spotted with the -parin root. All are injectible forms.

References

Drug Enforcement Administration. 2013. Controlled Substances Schedules. www.deadiversion.usdoj.gov

Epocrates Online. 2013. https://online.epocrates.com

FDA. 2008. Content and Forms of Labeling for Human Prescription Drug and Biological Products; Requirements for Pregnancy and Lactation Labeling. Federal Register 72 (104).

Lexi-Comp Inc. 2013. www.lexi.com

UpToDate. 2013. www.uptodate.com

INDEX

S

Z

Made in the USA
Lexington, KY
06 August 2014